The Pocket Guide to Key Terms for Hairdressing

Martin Green

Australia • Brazil • Japan • Korea • Mexico • Singapore • Spain • United Kingdom • United States

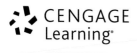
CENGAGE
Learning·

The Pocket Guide to Key Terms for Hairdressing
Martin Green

Publishing Director: Linden Harris

Publisher: Lucy Mills

Development Editor: Helen Green

Production Editor: Lucy Arthy

Editorial Assistant: Claire Napoli

Production Controller: Eyvett Davis

Marketing Executive: Lauren Mottram

Typesetter: MPS Limited, a Macmillan Company

Cover design: Adam Renvoize

For product information and technology assistance,
contact **emea.info@cengage.com**.
For permission to use material from this text or product,
and for permission queries, email **emea.permissions@cengage.com**.

This work is adapted from *Begin Hairdressing & Barbering 2e*, *Hairdressing: The Foundations 6e* and *Professional Hairdressing 6e*, published by Cengage Learning, Inc. © 2011.

British Library Cataloguing-in-Publication Data
A catalogue record for this book is available from the British Library.

ISBN: 978-1-4080-6041-4

Cengage Learning EMEA
Cheriton House, North Way, Andover, Hampshire, SP10 5BE United Kingdom

Cengage Learning products are represented in Canada by Nelson Education Ltd.

For your lifelong learning solutions, visit
www.cengage.co.uk

Purchase your next print book, e-book or e-chapter at
www.cengagebrain.com

Printed in Malta by Melita Press
1 2 3 4 5 6 7 8 9 10 – 14 13 12

Introduction to the Pocket Guide to Key Terms for Hairdressing

The vocabulary associated with hairdressing can be complicated and might seem daunting at first. This *Pocket Guide* aims to provide you with quick and simple definitions to all the key terms you will encounter throughout your studies.

The Pocket Guide to Key Terms for Hairdressing is designed to sit alongside our leading series of Hairdressing textbooks by Leo Palladino and Martin Green as a handy reference guide and easy-to-use revision tool.

Begin Hairdressing & Barbering: The Official Guide to Level 1, Revised Second Edition	*Hairdressing – The Foundations: The Official Guide to Level 2, Revised Sixth Edition*	*Professional Hairdressing: The Official Guide to Level 3, Revised Sixth Edition*
Martin Green	Martin Green and Leo Palladino	Martin Green and Leo Palladino
9781408039793	9781408039809	9781408039816
February 2011	February 2011	February 2011
£16.99	£24.99	£30.99

The revised QCF editions of the bestselling *Official Guides to Hairdressing at Level 1, 2 and 3* incorporate the latest changes to the hairdressing qualifications and are the only guides to hairdressing fully endorsed by Habia.

Buy your copies online now at **www.cengagebrain.com**.

A

Abrasion Broken, damaged skin (grazed).

Absorption The act of taking up or taking in water, e.g. a sponge absorbs water.

Accelerator A machine that produces radiant heat (infrared radiation) which can speed up chemical hair processes such as colouring or conditioning.

Accessories (hair) See ornamentation.

Accident book A record of accidents within the workplace required by health and safety law. Incidents in the accident book should be reviewed to see where improvements to safe working practices could be made.

Acid A substance that gives hydrogen ions in water and produces a solution with a pH below 7.

Acid conditioner A conditioner which has an acidic pH and helps to restore the hair's natural pH.

Acid mantle The layer of acidity maintained on the skin's surface which gives the skin slightly antiseptic properties.

Acne A condition causing spots to appear normally seen around the face, cheeks and mouth due to the overproduction of sebum from the sebaceous glands.

Activator A chemical used in bleaches or some perm lotions to start or boost its action.

Acute Sharp, severe or having pronounced symptoms.

Added hair A general term that covers the addition of hair pieces, wefts and extensions.

Adverse hair and scalp conditions Limiting factors that have an effect on what and how services are delivered to clients, e.g. head lice, psoriasis, alopecia, cysts, impetigo, scars, moles etc.

Aescalup Another name for thinning scissors.

African type hair Any hair type, which is tightly or loosely coiled, resembling black African hair.

Afro Describing an African-Caribbean hair type which has a tight curl formation.

Afro style A hairstyle effect that is produced by allowing tight, curly, hair to dry in a full, natural-dried way, lifting it outwards from the head to create a voluminous effect.

Aftershave balm Shaving balms that provide a moisturising effect that soothes and calms the skin after shaving. Moisturising balms are more suited for dry or sensitive skin types.

Aftershave lotion Moisturising lotions that replace lost oils and protect, cool and condition the skin after shaving. They are suitable for normal to dry skin types.

Aftercare advice Recommendations given to the client following a service to maintain the finished result and enable the benefits to be continued at home.

Albinism A condition of the hair and skin where there is an absence of pigment.

Albino The lack of any pigmentation within the skin and hair.

Alkali   A substance that gives hydroxide ions in water and produces a solution with a pH above 7.

Alkaline   A substance or compound having the qualities of an alkali.

Allergen   A substance that the skin is sensitive to and causes an allergic reaction.

Allergy   A sensitivity and possible intolerance to certain products, chemicals or compounds. See also patch test.

Aloe vera (shampoo ingredient)   A popular, mild natural base ideal for healthy hair and scalps that can be used on a frequent basis.

Alopecia   A general term covering a wide range of thinning or bald hair.

Alopecia areata   Small circular patches of baldness, which eventually grow back, or move to other areas.

Alopecia totalis   A term referring to the total lack of hair on the body.

Alpha keratin   Hair in its natural state, prior to styling, i.e. the state the hair is in before stretching and setting it into a new shape.

Ammonia   A strong smelling gas that is very soluble in water. An alkaline component of many high lift colours and ammonium based compounds found in bleach lighteners.

Ammonium thioglycolate   An active, alkaline substance in perm lotions that reacts with the disulphide bonds.

Anagen   The stage of hair growth during which the hair is actively growing.

Anatomy   The science of the structure of organic bodies.

Anchor   A beard shape that resembles an anchor from the centre of the bottom lip and around and up the chin.

Androgens   The name given to male hormones which can cause male pattern baldness.

Anaemia   The deficiency of red blood corpuscles or less than the normal quantity of haemoglobin in the blood.

Anhidrosis   The partial or complete absence of sweat secretion.

Anion   A negatively charged ion.

Anterior   Situated at the front.

Anti-dandruff treatment   A shampoo or conditioning treatment that is used to combat dandruff.

Anti-oxidant (conditioner)   A conditioner that stops the oxidation process of chemical services.

Antiseptic   A product which has the power to prevent the growth of bacteria.

Antiseptics   Substances that reduce the growth of micro-organisms that cause disease.

Apocrine gland   A type of sweat gland attached to the hair follicles in the armpits, pubic regions and nipples.

Appointment   An arrangement made for a client to receive a service on a particular date and at a particular time.

Appointment system   A system of organising the volume of work (client services or treatments) undertaken by a salon. This may be completed manually or by a computerized system.

Appraisal   A process of reviewing work performance over a period of time and planning future work objectives.

Arrector pili (muscle) The muscles that are attached to the walls of the follicle and, when contracted, raise the hair upright forming 'goose bumps'.

Artificial colour Any form of colour that is not a naturally occurring pigment. This is also called synthetic colour.

Aseptic The state of being free from germs.

Ash/ashen Hair colour shades that contain blue, violet tones producing 'cooler' effects.

Assessment An evaluation or judgement of input, value and/or attainment. Assessment techniques are used to evaluate the needs of the client.

Assessor A person qualified to judge the performance of a candidate.

Assignment A personal account or allocation of work. The account can be written, pictorial or practical and is based around clearly set objectives.

Astringent A substance which causes contraction and is applied after shaving to close the pores.

Asymmetrical Unevenly balanced, without an equal distribution of hair on either side.

Autoclave A device for sterilising items in high temperature steam.

Avant garde A genre of fashion that is considered progressive or exaggerated.

Awarding organisation An approved examining body such as City and Guilds, VTCT, Edexcel, OCR, who define the examinations and assessment processes and conduct the certification administration.

B

Bacillus Microscopic, rod-shaped forms of bacteria.

Backcombing/backbrushing Pushing hair back to bind or lift the hair using a comb or brush.

Backhand razoring A method of razoring where the cutting action occurs with a backhand technique.

Backwash A wash basin configuration where the client reclines backwards so that the neck rests in the basin.

Bacteria A tiny organism that can only be seen under a microscope.

Bactericide A substance which stops (kills) the growth of bacteria.

Baldness The loss of hair.

Banding An unwanted effect that appears as distinct bands of uneven colour.

Bantu knots Knots formed by twisting and curling a length of hair back on itself. The knots are often secured by a band if and where necessary.

Barrel curls A long hair dressing where wefts of hair are moulded into cylindrical shapes with an open centre. These are gripped into position and produce a chic, classic effect, popular for bridal work.

Barrel spring curl A type of pincurl with an open centre which produces an even curl effect. When formed, each loop is the same size as the previous one. It produces an even wave shape and may be used for reverse curling, which forms waves in modern hairstyles.

Barrier cream A cream that protects the skin against harmful moisture or infection.

Base An element (in chemistry) that combines with an acid to form a salt.

Baseline A cut section of hair which is used as a cutting guide for following sections of hair. The baselines will determine the perimeter of the hairstyle, or part of the style, and may take different shapes according to the effects required.

Basic uniform layer cut This type of haircut has sections that are equal i.e. the hair is the same length throughout.

BD Appointment abbreviation for blow dry.

Beard and moustache shapes For a beard: the facial hair shape around the mandible (jaw-line). For a moustache: any facial hair shape worn above the upper lip.

Beehive A hairstyle effect where long hair is backcombed and smoothed to create, tall, high shapes. This style was based on historical 'baroque' effects and was very popular and indicative of the 1960s.

Benefits Aspects that influence potential purchasers about the ways in which the functions of products or services may provide advantages for them.

Beta keratin The state the hair is in after it has been stretched and set into a new shape. See also alpha keratin.

Blackhead A whitish or yellowish spot at the surface of the skin, with a dark/blackish point. These spots are also known as comedones.

Bleach A hairdressing product that dissolves/removes natural colour pigments from hair. It is available in powder, cream and oil forms.

Blending A technique for mixing different colours of hair extension fibres to create more naturally occurring effects, multi-toned effects and highlighted effects.

Block colouring Creating a solid block(s) of colour on the hair. This can include stripes, veils, overlays, overlaps etc.

Blunt cutting Cutting sections of hair straight across (parallel) whilst holding the hair between the index and middle finger.

Body language Non-verbal communication provided by gestures, expressions and mannerisms that reveals the way a person is thinking or feeling.

Body odour (BO) The result of poor personal hygiene and lack of regular washing.

Bonding A method of attaching a hair weft using glue. It can be used for both hot and cold hair attachment systems.

Booster An activator or colour development accelerator.

Braid Another name for a plait or plaiting.

Brick cutting A way of point cutting into a held section of hair in different positions to create the 'scatter' pattern like brick work.

Brick wind A technique of winding rods into the hair so that there aren't any uniform divisions or 'roller marks' after the perm is finished. When the hair has been wound in this formation it looks like a brick wall.

Brilliantine   A cosmetic hair preparation for men that added shine and hold to hair; the classic, forerunner of contemporary waxes and glossers.

C

Calcium hydroxide   The chemical compound that is found in (no-lye) relaxers.

Camomile (shampoo ingredient)   The best ingredient for use on oily scalps as it has a natural lightening effect.

Cane rows   An effect created by multiple rows of scalp plaits that follow the contour of the head. Also known as corn rows.

Canities   Hair that is without pigment and therefore grey or white.

Cap highlights   A technique for highlighting hair where small sections or wefts of hair are drawn through a close fitting 'rubberised' cap and coloured or lightened. A convenient option for people who have a sensitivity to colouring and cannot have colour applied by other means.

Cap weave   A method of bonding hair onto a wig cap . Also known as a 'stocking foot'.

Capillary   A small 'hair-like' filament or tube, e.g. blood capillaries. These are the narrowest parts of the blood circulatory system that provide nourishment to the dermal papilla.

Case study   A study, examination or evaluation of specific factual or hypothetical events.

Catagen   The stage of hair growth during which the hair stops growing, but the hair papilla is still active.

Caustic   A very irritant substance, capable of burning or destroying tissue.

CBD   Appointment abbreviation for cut and blow dry.

Charge card   A form of payment where the complete amount of credit spent must be repaid by the cardholder each month to the card company.

Chemical reaction   A process of two or more chemicals combining to create a different substance.

Chemical sterilizers   A chemical solution or compound that will eradicate (kill) germs and bacteria that could be used to ensure tools and equipment are safe and hygienic.

Chemically treated hair   Hair that has been permed, coloured, bleached or relaxed.

Cheque   An alternative form of payment to that of using cash.

Chignon   A long 'hair-up' style forming a 'classic' knotted effect.

Chipping   A cutting technique where the points of the scissors are used to 'chip' in to sections of hair, removing small chunks to create texture.

Chronic   Long, continued or drawn out. The opposite of acute.

Cicatrical alopecia   Baldness due to scarring of the skin arising from chemical or physical injury. The hair follicle is damaged and permanent baldness results.

Clarifying shampoo   Strong, deep-acting shampoo often used prior to chemical services to remove the build-up of styling products and dirt.

Cleanser   Removes dead skin cells, sebum and debris from the skin.

Client care/customer care   A way of providing a service to customers that promotes goodwill, comfort, satisfaction and interest. Maintaining goodwill ultimately results in regular repeated business.

Client consultation   A service usually provided before the client has anything done to their hair to find out what the client wants, identify any styling limitations, provide advice and maintenance information and formulate a plan of action.

Clinical waste   Waste materials that have come into contact with body fluids, e.g. waste from ear-piercing must be collected and disposed of by special arrangements. The disposal of clinical waste is controlled by the Environment Agency.

Clip-on extensions   Pre-coloured wefts of hair that have clips or combs attached to them so that they can be affixed to the hair.

Clipper over comb   A technique of cutting hair with electric clippers, using the back of the comb as a guide. This technique is often used on very short hair and hairline profiles.

Clippers   Hair clippers are a mechanical cutting device operated by mains electricity or battery power. The cutting parts are created by two parallel blades with serrated teeth. The hand holds the direction of the clippers and subsequently, the cut. Hair is trapped within the teeth and the upper, moving blade oscillates back and forth to cut away all the hair that is exposed.

Clock-spring curl   A 'closed centre' pin curl.

Club cutting or clubbing hair   The most basic and most popular way of cutting sections of hair straight across (parallel) whilst holding the hair between the index and middle finger.

Coarse hair   A texture of hair where the individual thickness of the hair is greater than that of fine or medium types. Coarser hair has more layers of cuticle than those on finer types.

Coconut (shampoo ingredient)   Coconut contains an emollient which helps dry hair to regain its smoothness and elasticity.

Cohesive setting   The wetting, moulding and drying of hair into a stretched position. See also alpha keratin.

Coiffure   To arrange or dress hair.

Col (Rt or Fh)   Appointment abbreviation for colouring, either root application or full head.

Cold and hot bonded hair extensions   Cold bonding refers to a range of methods of connecting hair extensions to a client's natural hair without adding heat, e.g. with micro-rings, adhesive strips, adhesives. Hot bonding uses heat as the method for securing hair extensions to a client's natural hair, e.g. with glue sticks and resin based systems.

Cold-fusion hair extensions   A system of connecting hair extensions by using adhesives and adhesive strips.

Colour correction   An overarching term that encompasses a variety of colouring problems and processes, such as removing artificial colour, removing or correcting banded colour and re-colouring hair that has been lightened back to a depth and tone similar to the hair's natural pigmentation.

Colour star   See colour wheel.

Colour stripper   A colouring product that is specially formulated to reduce the size of synthetic or artificial pigments within a client's hair and therefore removing depth and tone from previously coloured hair.

Colour test   A diagnostic test to find out if a colour is suitable and/or achievable. It can be done by taking a test cutting or by applying colour on a small section of hair on the head.

Colour wheel   (Used during colour consultation.) A diagram made up of colours that provides an at-a-glance, visual aid for showing complementary colours and opposite, neutralising tones.

Colouring back   A colour correction process of re-colouring previously lightened hair back to the client's original, natural depth and tone. (Often requires pre-pigmentation.)

Comb twists   A twist created by a special comb that produces effects 'on' (and along) or 'off' the scalp.

Comb-out   The dressing of hair after the setting rollers have been removed using a brush or comb.

Comedones   A skin condition caused by the sebaceous glands. Appears as whitish or yellowish spots at the surface of the skin, with dark/blackish points.

Communication   Good communication is essential for establishing good customer service. We demonstrate this by listening to the client's requests, hearing and acting on what they are saying and always responding to clients in a polite but positive way.

Compatible   Able to mix without an unwanted reaction.

Complaints procedure   A formal, standardized approach adopted by the organisation to handle any complaints.

Compound henna   A mixture of vegetable henna and mineral elements that produce an incompatible hair dye. A contra-indication to all oxidation processes.

Concave   When referring to this in cutting terms, a concave shape has a perimeter that creates a curved shape which is higher at the centre rather than lower (i.e. convex).

Conditioner   A product that can be used to treat the hair or scalp, such as surface conditioners, penetrating conditioners, scalp treatments and leave-in conditioners.

Confidential information   Private or personal information, not intended for general discussion. This may include personal aspects of conversations with clients or colleagues, contents of client records, client and staff personal details (e.g. address, telephone numbers etc.), financial aspects of the business and hearsay/gossip.

Confidentiality   Client confidentiality is a discrete and professional way of handling client information without disclosing private matters to other staff or personnel.

Congenital hair loss/growth
Conditions that are present at birth and are caused by genetic factors. Inherited hair growth falls into normal congenital hair growth but there are other abnormalities which are rare and require medical treatment.

Congo plait A three-strand plait that starts, centrally, near the front hairline and continues closely to the scalp to the nape and continues as a freely hanging plait beyond. This is also known as French plait or Guinea plait.

Conjunctivitis An infectious, bacterial eye condition causing inflammation and redness.

Consumer and retail legislation Laws and regulations protecting people's purchasing rights.

Consumer Protection Act (1987) Legislation protecting customers from unlawful sales practices and mishandling of personal information. The Act safeguards the consumer from products that do not reach reasonable levels of safety.

Contact dermatitis A skin disorder caused by intolerance of the skin to the direct contact with a particular substance or a group of substances. On exposure to the substance the skin quickly becomes irritated and an allergic reaction occurs.

Contagious Communicable or transmissible (infectious).

Contaminate To infect with germs.

Continuing Professional Development (CPD) A title given to a process of updating knowledge and experience on a continuous basis within a particular vocational sector.

Contra-indication A limiting factor that affects the original/proposed plan of action, possibly allowing a treatment or service to continue, if and only when, specific conditions are met. In some cases a contra-indication will stop a proposed service altogether.

Contrasts A marked difference, e.g. between colours, say black and white.

Convex When referring to this in cutting terms, a convex shape has a perimeter that creates a curved shape which is lower (dips) at the centre. See also concave.

Corneum The stratum corneum or the horny layer of the skin.

Cornification The process of hardening e.g. the cornified layer of the skin is the area where maturing skin cells harden.

Cornrows/cornrowing A styling effect created by plaiting hair into small three stem plaits close to the scalp. Several corn rows produce linear or curved designs across the head.

Corrective colouring See colour correction.

Corrosive A substance that destroys organic tissue by chemical means.

Cortex The inner part of the hair where hairdressing chemical processes change or modify the natural hair, i.e. where permanent colour is deposited and where perms make physical changes to the hair.

COSHH An abbreviation for Control of Substances Hazardous to Health. COSHH safety regulations affect the way in which chemicals are handled at work. These health and safety regulations are created for your safety and must be adhered to.

Cowlick A hair growth pattern that appears at the front hairline where strong movement makes part of the hair stand away from the rest. This limits styling options and can be made worse by removing weight and length.

Credit card An alternative form of payment to using cash. These cards are held by those who have a credit account where there is a pre-arranged borrowing limit.

Crew cut A very short haircut where the hair length is even all over and shows the scalp.

Critical influencing factors Anything which could affect or limit the hairdressing service.

Croquignole A method of winding a curl from point to root.

Cross checking A final checking technique for assessing the continuity and accuracy of the hair cut. Where you find an imbalance in weight, or extra length that still needs to be removed, it provides you with the opportunity to remove it in order to create the perfect finish.

Cross-infection The passing on of disease (infectious micro-organisms) from one person to another either by contact or proximity. Cross-infection is caused by poor hygiene and sanitation.

Cross-infestation The transmission of animal parasites from one person to another.

Curtain rail A narrow band of hair that is left around the jaw-line.

Customer care See client care and communication.

Customer feedback The information retrieved by a variety of methods, used as a mechanism for evaluating the customer's experiences.

Cutaneous Relating/pertaining to the skin.

Cuticle The outer protective layers of the hair that produce an overlapped effect (like tiles on a roof).

Cutting angle The angle at which the scissors, razor etc. cuts the hair.

Cutting comb A type of comb that is between 12–20 cms long. It is used for general cutting and is rigid and parallel throughout its length or it is used for barbering and is tapered and more flexible. Most cutting combs have two different teeth patterns; one end finer with closer teeth for precision work or finer hair and the other end coarser with wider apart teeth for coarser hair and detangling.

Cysteine An amino acid containing a single sulphur atom. Two cysteines are oxidized to form a cystine molecule during the neutralising process of perming.

Cystine An amino acid containing a disulphide bond which occurs during perming when cystine is reduced to form two cysteine molecules.

D

Dandruff A commonly occurring skin dysfunction where there is an overproduction of epidermal cells. White scaling flakes are shed from the scalp and can be seen on the shoulder area of darker apparel. Dandruff is not contagious.

Data Protection Act   Legislation designed to protect the client's right to privacy and confidentiality. See also confidentiality.

Database   An archive or repository of information held on a computer, relating to business records including client and staff names, sales, products etc.

Debit card   A method of payment where the card authorizes immediate debit of the cash amount from the client's account.

Debris   A polite term referring to loose material that needs to be cleared away after different forms of styling, e.g. hair fragments, bands, glue, etc.

Decolouring   Removing synthetic colour from the hair. See also colour stripper.

Defining cream   A finishing product which gives control to unruly hair.

Defining wax   A finishing product that provides textural effects to short or long hair when used throughout the ends of the hair.

Demonstration   A display and explanation of a physical instruction.

Denman brush   A parallel, flat brush with removable cushioned bristles. It is used for general brushing, detangling hair before shampooing and drying straight hair of any length.

Density   The amount of hair follicles that populate a particular area of the skin or scalp.

Deodorant   A substance that removes or conceals offensive odours.

Depilation/depilatory effect   A process or substance that removes hair. Depilatory creams remove hair by chemical destruction.

Depth   The term used to describe the lightness or darkness of hair.

Dermatitis   A form of eczema which results in a red, sore, hot and itchy rash, usually between the fingers. This is known to be caused by contact with hairdressing chemicals and solutions. The condition is avoided by the wearing of PPE (such as disposable vinyl gloves).

Dermatologist   A (qualified) medical specialist for skin conditions.

Dermatology   The scientific study of the skin, its properties, features, dysfunctions, diseases and treatments.

Dermis   The lower layers of newer skin below the outer epidermis.

Detergent   A cleansing agent found in many washing materials and virtually all shampoos. It has a 'polar' molecule structure, where one end is attracted to dirt and grease and the other to water. When it comes into contact with dirt, it surrounds it and lifts it away from a surface, forming an emulsion.

Dexterity   The skill and ease of using the hands.

Diffuse   To scatter. This is often a term used when referring to sparsely populated or thinning hair.

Diffuse hair loss   A term relating to general thinning over the scalp.

Diffuser   An attachment for a blow-dryer which suppresses and disperses the blast of hot air and turns it into a multidirectional diffused heat.

Directional wind A technique of winding rods in so that, when finished, the hair will move in a particular direction.

Discolouration An incongruent colour effect which can result from poor colour application, incorrect colour choice, or can even indicate the presence of incompatibles.

Disconnection An area within a haircut where a continued style line is broken or disjointed. A deliberate and distinct difference exists creating two levels within the layering patterns or perimeter baselines.

Disease An abnormal condition affecting the body of an organism.

Disentangling The process of removing tangles and knots from hair. It is usually carried out with a wide tooth brush or detangling comb.

Disinfectant A chemical agent that will kill most germs and bacteria (unlike sterilisation which kills 100% of germs and bacteria) A typical example would be Barbicide™.

Disulphide bonds The chemical bonds within the hair that are permanently rearranged during perming, relaxing and neutralising.

Double-booking An error in the appointment system where clients' bookings overlap.

Double crown A common hair growth pattern which appears as two whorls of hair at, or around, the crown area. This feature limits styling options and will dictate how short and the direction of how the hair can be worn.

Double wind A variation of a weave wind where the hair left out of the rod is wound on another rod.

Dreadlocks A naturally occurring and permanent effect that occurs when hair locks together through mis-management and lack of grooming. It can also be aided by twisting tendrils of hair to create this matted effect.

Dressing The process of achieving finish to previously set hair.

Dry hair A condition in which the hair loses natural moisture levels affecting the handling, maintenance and style durability. It is often as a result of chemical treatments or heat styling.

Dry wax A non-greasy finishing product that provides textural effects to short or long hair when used throughout the ends of the hair.

E

Eczema A skin condition which appears as a reddening of the skin accompanied with itching and sometimes inflammation. It is thought to be associated with stress although one of its forms, dermatitis, can be triggered by contact with chemicals. See also dermatitis.

Effective communication Professional communication that is not ambiguous and provides clear instruction or information.

Effectiveness The quality of output achieved in a work setting.

Effleurage A light stroking massage movement applied with either the fingers or the palms of the hands and used during shampooing and conditioning.

Elasticity test A test to check the hair's ability to stretch and return to its normal length. This is a good indicator of the hair condition and strength of the internal structure of the hair.

Electricity at Work Regulations (1989) These regulations state that electrical equipment in the workplace should be tested every 12 months by a qualified electrician. The employer must keep records of the equipment tested and the date it was checked.

Electrolysis The destruction of hair by an electric current.

Emulsification During the removal of a root or full head application of permanent colour a little water is added to the colour to help release the residual product from the hair. This is then rinsed away before the shampoo process is conducted.

Emulsify In colouring terms, the process of adding a little water to the processed hair in order to loosen the colour from the hair, without adding detergent, before shampooing.

End papers Protective, paper wrapping, used around the points of the wound sections during perming to reduce/ eliminate the risk of 'fish hooks' i.e. buckled ends.

Enquiry A question presented by clients or business contacts to find out more information.

Environmental factors The effects caused or produced by UV damage, salt water and chlorine.

Epidermis The older, upper, protective layers of skin that constantly migrate towards the surface.

Epilation The extraction of hair.

Equal opportunities Non-discrimination on the basis of sex, race, disability, age, etc.

Erythma A reddening of the skin which is a result of an increased blood flow to the skin. It can be caused by infection, massage, electrical treatment, allergies, exercise or injury to the skin tissue.

Eumelanin Naturally occurring dark brownish or black pigments within the cortex of the hair.

Evacuation procedures The arrangements made by the salon for emergency purposes, e.g. exit routes, assembly points etc.

Excrete To separate and discharge waste matter from the blood, tissues, or organs.

Exfoliate To remove a layer of skin in flakes or scales.

Exfoliation The removal or shedding of a thin outer layer of skin from the epidermis. This is done by using a gentle abrasive substance to remove the surface skin.

External verifier (EV) A professional appointed by an awarding organisation to provide independent verification of the quality of assessment and quality assurance arrangements at centres approved to deliver nationally recognized qualifications.

F

Face or facial shapes   The size and shape of the facial bone structure. Face shapes include oval, round, square, heart, diamond, oblong and pear.

Fading (colour reference)   The loss of intensity of coloured hair due to harsh treatment, heat styling, wrong shampoos or environmental damage.

Fading (cutting reference)   A method of blending one graduated, layered area 'seamlessly' to another, within a haircut. Or graduating very short layers out and on to the skin, e.g. classic men's barbering where short hair is faded out on to the neck.

Feathering   A cutting term relating to a tapered or tapering effect.

Features   The aspects of a product or service that state its functions, i.e. what it does.

Finger waves   The process of moulding or styling hair in a pattern of alternating waves, using the fingers and a comb.

Fish hook   A point of hair that has been bent back during rollering or winding.

'Fish hooks'   A term used to describe the buckling at the points of the hair, due to incorrect winding during perming or styling.

Fish tail plait (herringbone plait)   A four strand plait which is achieved by crossing four pieces of hair over each other to create a 'herringbone' look.

Flat brush   A type of brush that has a handle that extends to the brush head with a flat and not curved profile. Flat brushes and paddle brushes are used for general brushing.

Flat twists   Where the hair is twisted and rolled by hand, flat to the scalp.

Follicle   A 'tube-like' indentation within the skin from which the hair grows.

Folliculitis   Inflammation of the hair follicles which may be caused by bacterial infection.

Forehand razoring   A method of razoring where the cutting action occurs with a forehand technique.

Fragilitis crinium   The technical term which is commonly known as split ends.

Franchise   A business which is licensed to operate under the branding and reputation of another.

Freehand cutting   A cutting technique carried out without holding the hair. This is usually to compensate for the natural fall of hair, e.g. cutting a fringe.

French plait   A three-strand plait that starts, centrally, near the front hairline and continues closely to the scalp to the nape and continues as a freely hanging plait beyond. This is also known as Congo plait or Guinea plait.

French pleat   A method of styling longer hair into a vertical roll positioned at the back of the head.

Friction (massage technique)   A firm, vigorous rubbing massage technique made by the fingertips and used during shampooing.

Full head application of colour or bleach   A colouring technique that requires a sequence of applications to the mid-lengths, ends and regrowth area.

Fungicide   A substance that stops the growth of, and kills fungi.

Furuncle A bacterial infection affecting the hair follicles and causing boils on the surface of the skin.

Fusing A method of attaching a micro strand of added hair to the natural hair with heat.

G

Gel weave A method of moulding the hair flat to the scalp using a gel. Then after completely drying the hair it forms a base on which to bond wefts of hair.

Germinal matrix The living part of the hair root where nutrients, carried in the blood supply, are converted into keratin (making hair and skin).

Germinative layer The growing or germinating layer of the skin.

Gift voucher A salon specific pre-payment method for treatments, services or retail sales.

Gland An organ that secretes something essential to the system or excretes waste material.

Goatee A narrow beard which circles the mouth and chin.

Goddess braids A form of extra-large corn rows/cane rows consisting of two to five corn rows/cane rows swept up on to the top of the head.

Goodwill An accounting term. The value of a business based on its reputation formed by the people who work for it.

Grade Attachment combs for clippers that provide a range of different, pre-defined cutting lengths.

Graduation A cutting technique that is created by a sloping variation which joins longer hair that over-falls shorter hair in one continuous, blended, cutting angle.

Greasy hair A condition caused by the over-production of natural oils, i.e. sebum, which exudes from glands within the scalp onto the surface and eventually the hair.

Grievance A cause for concern or complaint.

Grips and hair pins A variety of metal or plastic items for securing the hair into position.

Guideline The first or starting section of hair that is held and cut to the required length and then used as a template for the following sections.

Guinea plait A three-strand plait that starts, centrally, near the front hairline and continues closely to the scalp to the nape and continues as a freely hanging plait beyond. This is also known as Congo plait or French plait.

H

Hair (and skin) tests There are a number of tests that can be carried out prior to a service to help evaluate the effects of processing upon the hair and skin. These tests could reveal contra-indications to services or provide information on how the hair can be processed under certain conditions, e.g. porosity test, elasticity test, skin test, pull test etc.

Hair bulb The lower club-shaped part of the hair that is attached to the germinal matrix.

Hair colour   The resultant effect from two colour aspects within the hair. These are depth (the lightness or darkness of a colour) and tone (the degree of red, gold, ash etc.).

Hair extensions   Pieces of artificial or natural hair that are added either, temporarily or for a longer period, to a client's natural hair to provide instant length, volume or movement.

Hair growth patterns   These are double crown, widows peak, cow lick, nape whorl, natural parting and regrowth.

Hair shaft   The portion of hair that projects above the epidermis.

Hair tendency   Refers to a hair's straightness, wave, body, or curl.

Hair texture   Refers to the thickness or thinness of individual hairs, either coarse, medium or fine.

Hair trap   A flexible nylon or plastic plug that helps to stop hair from entering the drain

Hairdressing and Beauty Industry Authority (HABIA)   HABIA is part of the Consumer Services Industry Authority (CSIA) and is the standards setting body responsible for National Occupational Standards in hairdressing and beauty therapy.

Hairspray   A fixative originally derived from shellac, now made from water soluble compounds and is also known as lacquer.

Halitosis   Bad breath.

Hamilton classification   The scale that defines the different stages of male hair loss.

Hard water   Water containing minerals which do not easily lather. Hard water contains magnesium and calcium salts.

Harmonizes   Goes with or complements.

Harmony   Maintaining a good working relationship and atmosphere with your fellow staff.

HASAWA   The abbreviated term referring to the Health and Safety at Work Act (1974).

Hazard   Something with a potential to cause harm.

Head lice   An infestation of animal parasites. A very contagious contra-indication. The trichological term for head lice is pediculosis capitis.

Health and Safety (First Aid) Regulations (1981)   Legislation that states that workplaces must have appropriate and adequate first-aid provision.

Health and Safety at Work Act   Legislation that lays down the minimum standards of health, safety and welfare requirements in all workplaces.

Heat protection spray   Used in conjunction with electrically heated styling tools. The product laminates the outer layer of the hair so that it is protected from the damaging effects of heat.

Heated rollers   Used for dry setting techniques. These are electrically heated rollers that are used as an alternative to wet setting. Heated rollers produce softer results than wet setting.

Heated tongs   An item of heat styling equipment that provides movement, lift, volume, waves or spiralled curls on dry hair.

Henna A natural colourant derived from the Lawsonia plant. Its leaves are mixed with water to create a red hair dye.

Herpes simplex The scientific name for cold sores.

Hi-lites/highlights A term for a very popular partial colouring technique, where small sections of natural hair are isolated (with foil, wraps, meche etc.) and coloured or lightened to give a multi-toned effect.

Hirsutism A condition that causes excessive hair growth in women.

HL or H/L Appointment abbreviation for highlighting.

HL T sect Appointment abbreviation for highlight, top and sides only.

Holding angle The angle at which the hair is held out from the head when completing a haircut.

Holding tension The even pressure applied to a section of hair when it is held ready for cutting.

Hood dryer An electrical item that applies dry heat to the head by sitting beneath it. The heat is adjustable and the timer can be preset to enable previously wet set hair to be dried.

Hopscotch winding A perming technique for partially processing alternative sections/meshes of hair, whilst leaving the others sections out. This produces a multi-textural effect.

Hot towels These towels are heated and used in barbering for shaving services.

Hot-bonded hair extensions A system of connecting hair extensions by using resin or hard plastics.

Humectant A hygroscopic substance attracting water or locking moisture into the hair.

Humidity The level of moisture in the air.

Hydrogen peroxide An oxidising agent used in many hairdressing processes. It readily gives off oxygen in chemical reactions, developing or processing colours lighteners etc.

Hydrophilic A term used in reference to the 'polar' detergent molecule. The hydrophilic end is and attracted to water.

Hydrophobic A term used in reference to the 'polar' detergent molecule. The hydrophobic end is repelled by water and is therefore attracted to grease.

Hygroscopic Something that absorbs moisture from the atmosphere.

I

ICC (International Colour Chart) system A tabular system for identifying hair colours made by different manufacturers by their depth and tone.

Immerse To dip into a liquid.

Impetigo A very contagious bacterial infection of the epidermal layers of the skin. It is usually identified as large brownish scabs around the mouth and cheeks. This contra-indication must be referred to a GP.

Incompatibility Refers to incompatible chemistry. When 'inorganic' compounds are present within the hair for example colour restorers, 'Just for Men' or compound henna. They will be incompatible with organic based chemicals made from carbon, hydrogen and oxygen (e.g. hydrogen peroxide).

Incompatibility test A method of testing hair to see if previous chemical treatments are compatible with those used with professional salons.

Incompatible Causing a chemical reaction on mixing; as between a chemical being added to the hair and another chemical already on the hair.

Infection The communication of disease from one body to another. An infection is the colonization of a host organism by a parasite species.

Inflammation Swelling, heat and pain. Inflammation is a process by which the body's white blood cells and chemicals protect us from infection and foreign substances such as bacteria and viruses.

Influencing factors Anything which could affect the hairdressing service.

Ingrowing hair A painful condition where a build-up of skin occurs at the upper end of the hair follicle, causing the hair to grow under the surface of the skin.

Internal verifier (IV) An approved centre's staff who is responsible for ensuring that the assessment process has been conducted in a way to meet the quality assurance criteria of the awarding organisation.

Inversed clippering A way of holding the clippers to produce outlines, necklines and detail within a design.

Inversion A term used in cutting to describe a "V" shape within a layering pattern or perimeter outline.

Irritant An agent that induces irritation.

J

Job description A documented set of written details pertaining to a person's specific job role, duties and responsibilities.

Jojoba (shampoo ingredient) A natural base better on normal to drier hair types.

Jumbo comb A large, wide tooth comb used for detangling hair or evenly applying conditioner to wet hair.

K

Keratin The protein that makes up the chemical composition of hair, nails and skin.

Knots The effect produced when long hair is wound, positioned and secured to take on a tied or knotted rope like effect.

L

Lacquer A fixative originally derived from shellac, now made from water soluble compounds and commonly known as hairspray.

Lanugo A down-like, fine hair.

Lathering The initial process of applying lather to a client's face to help soften bristles prior to wet shaving.

Lawsonia A 'leaf' extract used for making henna from the Egyptian privet shrub.

Layering (layered cut) A cutting technique carried out on either short or long hair to produce a multi-length effect.

Legal requirements The laws affecting the way businesses are operated, how the salon or workplace is set up and maintained, people in employment and the systems of working which must be maintained.

Legislation Laws created by parliament.

Lemon (shampoo ingredient) Contains citric acid ideal for oily scalp types or for removing product build-up.

Lesion An injury, wound or abnormal area of tissue on the body.

Lighteners Products that remove natural tone from the hair such as bleach or high lift colour.

Limits of your authority The extent of your responsibility at work.

Linear patterns Patterns created from either straight or curving lines or a combination of both.

Lip-line moustache A narrow lined moustache.

Litmus A water-soluble mixture of different dyes extracted from lichens.

Litmus paper A pH indicator made up from a treated paper strip with litmus. It is used to find out if something is an acid (turning blue litmus paper red) or an alkali (turning red litmus paper blue.)

Litmus test A test for chemical acidity or basicity (alkalinity) using litmus paper.

Long hair graduation A cut when the inner/upper layers of a haircut are shorter than the lengths of the outline, perimeter hair.

Long-lasting colour See quasi-permanent colour.

Low-lights A colouring effect where sections of hair are woven and placed into meche, foil, packets etc. using colour instead of bleach/lighteners.

Lubricant Making oily or slippery.

Ludwig A scale defining different stages of female hair loss.

Lye (and no-lye) A term referring to the chemical composition of relaxing treatments (i.e. sodium hydroxide based or not).

M

Male pattern baldness (MPB) A type of alopecia caused by sensitivity to androgens (male hormones).

Management of Health and Safety at Work Regulations (1999) Legislation requiring employers to make formal arrangements for maintaining a safe, secure working environment under the Health and Safety at Work Act. This includes staff training for competently monitoring risk in the workplace, known as a risk assessment.

Manual Handling Operations Regulations (1992) Legislation requiring employers to carry out a risk assessment of all activities which involve manual handling (lifting and moving objects) with the aim being to prevent injury due to poor working practice.

Manufacturer's instructions Stated guidance issued by manufacturers or suppliers of products or equipment, concerning their safe and efficient use.

Materials A variety of items other than tools and equipment for carrying out work including colouring packets, foils, wraps, meche etc.

Medicated shampoo Helps to maintain the normal state of the hair and scalp. Medicated shampoo contains antiseptics such as juniper or tea tree oil.

Medulla The central part of the hair that is only found in coarser hair types.

Melanin The naturally occurring pigments formed within the skin and hair.

Melanocytes Cells that produce melanin within the skin.

Merchandize Goods, products and equipment for sale.

Metallic dye A hair colour containing metallic salts.

Mexican moustache A moustache following the line of the upper lip and extends around and down towards the chin.

Microbes Living organisms of very small size.

Microorganisms Living organisms, bacteria etc. of microscopic size.

Mint (shampoo ingredient) A natural base suited to normal to slightly oily scalps, often used as a frequent use shampoo.

Moisturisers Products adding moisture to the hair.

Moisturising balms Cooling, soothing and moisture replenishing lotions applied after shaving to counteract the abrasive effects of the process.

Monilethrix The technical term that describes a rare condition that under a microscope looks like the hair is 'beaded', i.e. thicker and thinner areas of hair along the hairshaft due to uneven cellular production.

Mood board A collection of ideas, themes, textures, colours etc. that form the basis of a design plan, e.g. a competition mood board.

Moulding clay A dual purpose product for styling or finishing that bonds the hair with a firm hold. It is used on most hair lengths to give a firm textural bond.

N

Nape The back (posterior) part of the neck.

Nape whorls A hair growth pattern which affects shorter, cut hairstyles. The nape hair grows inwards, towards the centre of the back, rather than downwards. This is a limiting factor for some hairstyles.

National Occupational Standards (NOS) The standards defined by an industry for different levels of ability covering all the tasks and processes involved in the industrial sector.

Natural hair Hair that still has its original, natural structure.

Neck brush A small hand brush with very flexible bristles for clearing debris away from the client's face, neck etc. during and after styling.

Neck wool A continuous 'sausage-like' length of cotton wool used during perming (and other services) to protect the client from spillages and debris.

Neutralizer The chemical that is applied after perming and rinsing, which re-balances and fixes the hair into its new shape.

Nine-section wind A classic technique for perming that starts by sectioning and securing the hair into nine, pre-defined workable areas.

Nit The egg casing containing the larvae of immature, head lice (pediculosis capitis).

Non-conventional styling materials Items that can be used to style hair other than rollers and pin clips such as rags, buttons, chopsticks, straws, rik-rak etc.

Non-verbal communication Communicating using body language, such as using your eyes, face and body to transmit your feelings.

Normalising products Post-relaxing treatments and shampoos. They are also referred to as 'stabilizers' or 'neutralising' products for the relaxing process.

NVQ An abbreviation for National Vocational Qualification. These are job-ready qualifications at a range of different levels.

O

Oblong facial shape An outline perimeter facial shape that has proportions that roughly resemble an oblong shape.

Occipital bone The protruding part at the back of the head (cranium) that provides contour and shaping to shorter cut layered hairstyles.

Off-base The positioning of a roller so that it doesn't sit on its own base. Creates end movement without volume and lift at the root area.

Oil (shampoo ingredient) Can contain a range of natural bases such as pine, palm and almond. These are used to smooth and soften drier hair and scalps.

Oily scalp A condition caused by the over-production of natural oils, i.e. sebum, which exudes from glands within the scalp on to the surface and eventually the hair affecting its handling, maintenance and style durability.

On-base The positioning of a roller so that it sits squarely on its own 'footprint' area to create end curl and root lift/ volume.

One-length hair cut A cutting technique where all the hair is cut with the natural hair fall to produce a one-length effect, i.e. the classic 'bob'.

Open (cut throat) razor A razor that has a fixed, rigid blade that folds into its handle for safety. The blade is kept keen (sharp) by regular stropping and honing. The razor must be sterilized before each use.

Organic A substance that contains the chemical element carbon and relates to living (or once living) sources.

Ornamentation The term refers to the accessorising of hair with enhancements, e.g. jewellery, beads, ribbons, tiaras, decorative pins/grips etc.

Outlines The shapes created by the perimeter of nape and front hairlines.

Oval facial shape An outline perimeter facial shape that has proportions that roughly resemble an oval or elliptical shape.

Overbooking An error in the appointment system where clients' bookings overlap.

Oxidation A chemical reaction where oxygen is added to a substance or compound during the chemical process.

P

Paddle brush See flat brush.

Papilla The lower part of the follicle where living cells migrate upwards producing hair growth.

Para-dyes A term that refers to permanent colours containing para-phenylenediamine or PPD.

Para-phenylenediamine (PPD) A dye compound found in many permanent colours.

Parasite An animal or vegetable living upon or within another organism.

Partial colouring A term that applies to areas of the head and could include techniques such as slices, block colour, polishing/shoe shining, woven or pull through highlights and lowlights etc.

Partial relaxing Chemical relaxers are only applied to parts of the hair, e.g. at the nape area.

Pathogen A pathogen or a biological agent that causes disease or illness to its host.

Pediculosis capitis The trichological term for the head louse. An infestation of animal parasites. A very contagious contra-indication. See also nit.

Pencil moustache A narrow shape following the natural line of the upper lip.

Penetrating conditioner A name given to a group of deeper acting conditioners that work on the inner cortex of the hair.

Perm (permanent wave) A two-part system for adding movement to hair by chemical means.

Perm solution The first part of a permanent wave system which chemically modifies the hair's inner structure.

Permanent tint/colour A penetrating colour product that adds synthetic pigments to natural hair until it grows out.

Personal development Recognising the opportunities that arise at work when you get the chance to learn new things.

Personal development plan An on-going action plan for self-improvement that defines personal objectives or targets set over a period of time and often reviewed during an appraisal.

Personal presentation Professional personal presentation can refer to, personal health and hygiene, the use of personal protective equipment, clothing and accessories suitable for salon work.

Personal protective equipment (PPE) This health and safety term refers to all of the items of personal equipment that are supplied by the employer for employees' safety such as gloves, aprons etc.

Personal Protective Equipment (PPE) at Work Regulations (1992) Legislation requiring employers to identify, through risk assessment, those activities which require special protective equipment to be worn or used. Instruction should be provided on how the personal protective equipment should be used or worn in order to be effective.

Personalising A term which refers to a variety of cutting techniques applied to a style dependent on the client's specific needs.

Petrissage A slower circulatory kneading massage movement of the skin that lifts and compresses underlying structures of the skin. This movement is generally used for a scalp massage when applying conditioner.

pH The presence of positive hydrogen ions with a compound which denotes its levels of acidity or alkalinity.

pH balance The natural acid mantle of skin and hair at pH5.5.

pH level A measurement of a solution that denotes whether it is alkaline (pH 8–14), or acid (pH 6–1). A neutral solution is pH 7.

Pharaoh A beard that projects from the base of the chin.

Pheomelanin A naturally occurring hair pigment that is yellowish or golden in colour.

Piggy back wind A technique of winding curlers or rods into the hair to create a multi-textured effect that has curls and movement of differing diameters.

Pigment A granular form of colouration that can be natural or artificial.

Pityriasis Commonly refers to flaking (or scaling) of the skin.

Pityriasis capitis A granular form of colouration that can be natural or artificial.

Pleat A visual description of hair that is folded, such as a French pleat.

Point cutting A cutting technique where the cutting angle is changed to remove hair bulk from the ends of each cutting section.

Pointing See point cutting.

Porosity The speed at which hair absorbs (and retains) moisture.

Porous hair Hair that has lost surface protection and therefore has a greater absorption and less resistance to chemicals and products. This affects the hair's manageability, handling and ability to hold in a style.

Portfolio A system for recording experiences, case studies, personal accounts, results from tests or assessments and the findings from projects and assignments.

Post-damping The term referring to the application of perming lotion to previously wound curlers.

Posterior Situated at the back.

Postiche A dressed hairpiece.

Post-perm/colour treatment A conditioning treatment that is applied after processing to add shine, improve strength and close the cuticles.

Posture The positioning of the body. Good posture is when the body is in alignment. Correct posture enables you to work longer without becoming tired. It prevents muscle fatigue (tiredness) and stiff joints.

Potentially infectious condition A medical condition or state of health which may be transmitted to others. See also cross-infection.

Practise block A training head or modelling head that can be used to practise hairdressing techniques and styling effects.

Pre-damping The application of perming lotion prior to winding in the curlers.

Pre-perm treatment A product applied to the hair before perming to balance out uneven porosity.

Pre-pigmentation The preparatory process of adding warm tones to pre-lightened hair when (and before) reintroducing depth. This counteracts the unwanted effects that will often appear if this process is not carried out first, e.g. green hues.

Pre-softening A process of softening resistant white hair with hydrogen peroxide.

Pressing A thermal styling technique using a heated metal pressing comb to straighten the hair.

Prices Act (1974) The price of products has to be displayed in order to prevent a false impression to the buyer.

Productivity The levels of output achieved in a work context.

Professional advice Providing information based upon experience and knowledge.

Project Private study focusing upon a set topic or object. See also assignment.

Provision and Use of Work Equipment Regulations (PUWER) (1998) Regulations laying down the ways in which work equipment must be used safely.

Psoriasis Non-infectious areas of thickening skin/epidermal layers usually around the elbows and knees.

Public liability insurance A compulsory insurance protecting employees, customers and visitors against the consequences of personal injury.

Pull test This tests the hair's ability to stay within its follicle. For example a pull test done before a hair extensions service will indicate how well the hair will be able to take the extra weight of added hair.

PW Appointment abbreviation for permanent wave (perm).

Q

Quasi-permanent colour A colour that is mixed with a low-strength developer to create a longer-lasting effect. This treatment does show a regrowth and does need a skin test 24–48 hours prior to the service.

R

Radial brush A completely round brush. The inner body of the brush is usually metal allowing the brush to heat up. It is used for blow-drying with volume, lift, wave and curl on short and long length hair.

Reagent A substance that initiates (brings about) a chemical reaction.

Real hair extensions A variety of different quality extensions made from human hair. These are usually chemically processed although more expensive hair extensions can be bought in a natural, unprocessed state.

Rearranger An ammonium thioglycolate based compound used to pre-soften tight, curly hair prior to perming.

Record cards Confidential cards recording the personal details of each client registered at the salon. These cards also record services a client received and retail product purchases. The information may be stored electronically on the salon's computer.

Reducing agent A product that releases hydrogen into the hair such as colour strippers, de-colour, perm lotion.

Referral (client) The situations where you need to redirect clients to other sources of treatment or service, i.e. when there are adverse hair and skin conditions, or because of other services that your salon doesn't provide.

Regrowth The band of natural hair growing back at the root area (12.5mm per month) which will require some form of processing to match the mid lengths and ends.

Relaxer/relaxing A chemical process (usually in two parts) which removes natural movement/curl from the hair.

Removal solution A chemical formulated to dissolve the adhesive connecting the hair extension to the hair in cold-fusion systems.

Removal tool A pair of metal pliers used for breaking the bond connecting the hair extension to the hair in hot-bonded systems.

Repetitive strain injury (RSI) Injury incurred through repetition of movement of a particular part of the body.

Resale Prices Act (1964 and 1976) The manufacturers can supply a recommended retail price (MRRP), but the seller is not obliged to sell at the recommended price.

Reshape/reshaping Cutting hair back into style. A six-weekly reshape cut will maintain a hairstyle.

Resources The variety of means available to a business that can be utilized or employed within any given task or project including time, money, staff, equipment, stock, etc.

Responsible persons A health and safety term referring to the person(s) at work to whom you should report any issues, problems or hazards. E.g. a supervisor, line manager or your employer.

Restructurant A deep acting treatment that will help to re-strengthen natural hair.

Restyle Cutting hair into a new style.

Revenue stream A source of income that comes into a business, e.g. retail sales, sales of services, sales of treatments etc.

Reverse graduation A cutting technique that joins together shorter hair down to longer hair in one continuous cutting angle.

RIDDOR Reporting of Injuries, Diseases and Dangerous Occurrences Regulations. This legislation requires the employer to report certain injuries or diseases occuring in the workplace.

Ringworm A fungal disease also known as tinea capitis. It is a very contagious contra-indication and must be referred to a GP.

Risk The likelihood of harm occurring from a potential hazard.

Risk assessment A process of looking for and assessing the hazards within the workplace.

Role play A way of exploring different scenarios by simulation.

Roll A visual description of hair that is rolled to create a bulked, rounded shape. This can be aided by using a 'bun ring' or similar styling aid.

Rollers A variety of circular formers of differing diameters used for setting hair when dry (e.g. Velcro self-cling) or wet (e.g. 'Skelox').

Rooftop moustache A shape that extends from under the nose to form a straight 'chevron' or inverted 'V' shape.

Root lift mousse A mousse that has a directional nozzle allowing you to apply foam at or near to the roots. It is used on hair that needs body.

Root perm A technique for winding perming rods near the root area to produce lift without end movement.

Rotary massage A quicker and firmer circular movement used during the shampooing process.

Round facial shape An outline perimeter facial shape that has proportions that roughly resemble a circular or round shape.

S

Safety razor A hand-held razor that is fitted with disposable blades providing a more convenient, hygienic option, as the blades can be replaced for each client.

Sale and Supply of Goods Act (1994) The vendor must ensure that the goods they sell are of satisfactory quality and reasonably fit. The goods must be the standard that would be regarded by a reasonable person as satisfactory having taken into account the description of the goods, the price and other relevant circumstances. The vendor must ensure that the goods can meet the purpose they are claimed to do.

Salon policy The hairdressing procedures or work rules issued by the salon management.

Salon requirements The hairdressing procedures or work policies issued by the salon management.

Salon services The extent and variety of all the services offered in your workplace.

Scabies The common name of the itch mite. This animal parasite burrows beneath the surface of the skin and is very highly contagious. Referral to a GP is essential.

Scalp The skin covering the top of the head.

Scalp plaits Also known as a French plait, a cane row or corn row.

Scissor over comb A technique of cutting hair with scissors, using the back of the comb as a guide. This technique is usually used when the hair is at a length that cannot be held between the fingers.

Scrunch drying A form of finger drying technique, where the lengths of the hair are dried (often with the aid of a diffuser) and compacted/crushed by the fingers to maximize the hair's natural movement.

Sculpting A technique describing a range of 3D shapes created within a haircut.

Sebaceous cyst A swelling of the oil gland within the hair follicle.

Sebaceous glands Sack-like appendages on the sides of the follicle that secrete sebum onto the hairshaft.

Seborrhea An overproduction of natural oils causing a greasy scalp and hair.

Sebum A natural oil produced by the sebaceous gland.

Self-adhesive extensions Pre-coloured wefts of hair that have self-cling, peel-off strips that reveal a sticky tape that attaches the extension to the client's hair.

Semi-permanent colour A semi-permanent colour is not mixed with hydrogen peroxide. It only penetrates to the lower cuticle and therefore lasts for a few washes.

Senegalese twists A twisting technique that resembles the plaited effect created by cornrows.

Sensitized hair Fragile hair that has been sensitized by previous chemical or mechanical processes, e.g. bleached, high lights, heat styled etc.

Serum A silicone based product that is used as a finishing product to smooth the hair and to add shine.

Shape, proportion and balance The physical and notional aspects that control hair design and hairstyling.

Shaper razor A type of razor with disposable blades that is used for cutting and styling hair, but not for shaving. It therefore has uses for both women's and men's hairstyling.

Sharps/ sharps box A term to describe sharp objects e.g. razors and razor blades, scissors. A sharps box is a designated sealed container used for the safe disposal of sharp items, e.g. used razor blades.

Shaving cream Moisturises the skin whilst providing a good lubricant for shaving. Moisturising shaving creams can be used for all skin types, but normal to drier skins will benefit most from the creams.

Shaving oil Contains natural plant oils that moisturise the face whilst providing the perfect base for a close, comfortable shave. They are particularly suited to those with sensitive skins.

Shaving soap Provides the basic lubrication for a good close shave. Moisturising shaving soaps will create a rich, lubricating lather that softens and moisturises the skin.

Short graduation cut A short graduation cut is when the inner and upper layers of a haircut are longer than the lengths of the outline, perimeter hair.

Skin test A test done prior to colouring to establish whether a client has a sensitivity or reaction to chemical products.

Slicing A texturising technique for cutting hair using the sharp blades of scissors without opening and closing them, like using a razor or shaper.

Slicing (colouring) Sections of colour placed in the hair to bring attention to style lines or styling features.

Slider cutting A technique used with very sharp scissors assimilating the action and effect produced by razoring to create a tapering effect.

Sodium bromate An oxidising agent found in colouring products.

Sodium Laureth Sulphate (SLS) A commonly used detergent compound found in shampoos.

Soya (shampoo ingredient) Helps to lock in moisture for the hair and scalp.

Spiral setting A wind from root to point along a cylindrical rod or roller to create cascading curls.

Spiral wind A perming technique of winding longer hair from root to point.

Split ends A condition of the hair where a damaged cuticle exposes the inner cortex of the hair allowing it to split along its length (fragilitas crinium).

Square facial shape An outline perimeter facial shape that has proportions that roughly resemble a square shape.

Steamer An item of salon equipment that is used for accelerating the development time of bleach lighteners. It produces a moist heat which stops the bleach drying out during the lightening process.

Sterile Free from germs.

Sterilisation The complete eradication of living bacteria and germs.

Stock check An accounting process for monitoring and controlling the movements and usage of stock.

Stock rotation When shelves are re-stocked the newer product is put at the back and the older stock is brought to the front to be sold first.

Storyboard A way of pictorially and verbally collating ideas and concepts into a visual flow chart or schedule of events.

Straightener (chemical) An ammonium-based lotion similar to perms that can be used to remove wave in hair.

Straightening Reducing the curl or wave in hair.

Strand test A test carried out upon hair prior to chemical services to determine the effects of processing.

Strengths and weaknesses The difference between personal skill areas that you excel in and those that you need to work on.

Style line The directions in which the hair is positioned or appears to flow.

Styling mousse A general styling aid for adding volume and providing hold when blow-drying or setting.

Stylist Another name for a qualified hairdresser or hairstylist.

Subcutaneous layer/tissue A fatty layer of cells at the lower dermis beneath the skin.

Sudoriferous Producing sweat.

Surface conditioner A light conditioner that works on the outside of the hair to smooth and fill areas of damaged, missing or worn cuticle until the next shampoo.

Surfactant A surface acting chemical detergent that cleanses the surface of the hair and skin.

Sweat A clear, salty liquid produced by glands in the skin that helps to regulate body temperature.

Sweat gland Small tubes in the skin of the dermis and epidermis which excrete sweat. Their function is to regulate body temperature through the evaporation of sweat from the skin's surface.

Sycosis An inflammatory disease affecting the follicles, particularly the beard. Appearing as pustules or papules, perforated by the hair.

Symmetrical Balanced by means of an even and equal distribution of hair on either side.

Synthetic colour Any form of colour that is not a naturally occurring pigment. A term that is often used instead of artificial colour.

Synthetic fibre extensions A range of alternative, fibrous materials used for extending hair (nylon, acrylic, Kerakalon etc.).

Systemic hair loss/hair growth Systemic hair loss is caused by a defect in one of the body systems or organs e.g. the heart. Normal systemic hair growth is caused by changes in hair growth associated with puberty, pregnancy and menopause. Abnormal systemic includes excessive hair growth and partial or total hair loss.

T

T liner A type of clipper with a different blade type to standard clippers, enabling closer cut outlines around ears, necklines and facial hair shapes.

T section highlights A partial highlighting technique around the hairline and along the parting only.

Tail or pin comb A comb that provides tension when combing through sections and helps to manage hair. It is used for sectioning hair into workable sizes depending on the setting, plaiting or twisting technique used.

Tapered necklines Soft outlines that follow the natural hairline shape so that the nape outline appears to fade out with no harsh lines visible.

Tapering Cutting a hair section by removing thickness towards the ends of the hair to form a tapered point, i.e. a point like that of a sharpened pencil.

Tapotement A brisk tapping or slapping massage movement which is also known as percussion.

Tariff A displayed list of fixed charges.

Tea tree oil (shampoo ingredient) A natural essential oil, like an antiseptic, which will fight infections on the scalp.

Telogen The period during which a hair ceases to grow before it is shed.

Temporal Bones which form the lower sides of the head.

Temporary bonds The hydrogen bonds within the hair that are modified and fix the style into shape.

Temporary colour Colour added to hair that lasts until the next wash.

Tensile strength test A test that will determine the breaking point of a hair. This relates directly to the internal structure of the hair within the cortex.

Tension The state of being stretched.

Terminal hair The coarser type of hair that is found on the scalp and other areas of the body. There are three specific stages of terminal hair growth anagen, telogen and catagen.

Texturising A variety of cutting techniques that are used to achieve different effects within the cutting scheme of a hairstyle.

Thinning A way of reducing the thickness or amount of hair without having an effect on the overall (apparent) hair length. Techniques would include razoring, texturising or by using thinning scissors.

Thinning scissors Scissors which will remove uniform bulk from any point between the root area and ends.

Tinea capitis A fungal disease commonly known as ringworm. It is a very contagious contra-indication and must be referred to a GP.

Tinting back A colour correction process of re-colouring previously lightened hair back to the client's original, natural depth and tone.

Tone Refers to the tonal (the colour) properties of hair. These are grouped into reds, golds, mahogany, ash, chestnut etc.

Toner/toning Adding pastel colours to previously, lightened hair to control the final desired effect. Toning can neutralize unwanted tones or add depth or colour to hair that is too light.

Tonging A technique of styling hair with heated equipment. The tongs are cylindrical in shape and, when heated, hair is wound around and held in place for a few seconds and then released.

Total look A term that is often used to describe a visual themed effect that incorporates hair, clothes, accessories and make-up.

Traction alopecia An area of baldness that is caused by the excessive pulling of hair at the root. It is often associated with longer hair worn in plaits, twists, hair-ups and extensions.

Trades Descriptions Act (1968 and 1972) Products must not be falsely or misleadingly described in relation to their quality, fitness, price or purpose, by advertisements, orally, displays or descriptions. Since 1972 it is also a requirement to label a product clearly, so that the buyer can see where the product was made.

Tramliner A specialist clipper with a tapered, narrow blade for detailing designs on the hair.

Trichologist A professionally qualified person who specializes in the diagnosis and treatment of hair and scalp problems.

Trichology The scientific study and treatment of hair, its properties, diseases and dysfunctions.

Trichorrexis nodosa A condition where the hair has damaged sites of cuticle allowing the fibrous cortex to break through. This makes the hair weakened, very knotted and hard to manage.

Trichosiderin An iron-containing pigment found in human red hair.

Trichotillomania The technical term given to a nervous disorder where one is obsessed with pulling out one's own hair.

Triethanolamine Laureth Sulphate (TLS) A surfactant detergent used in cleaning products.

Trim (trimming hair) A trim denotes a haircut where very little is taken off in order to maintain a hairstyle. Typically a six-weekly reshape is another name for a trim.

Twist A technique of styling hair, or multiple stems of hair, by twisting them together.

U

Ultraviolet radiation (UV) A form of sterilisation carried out in salons by putting tools and equipment into a UV cabinet.

Uniform layer cut This type of haircut has sections that are equal, i.e. the same length throughout.

Unit of competence The smallest unit that can be separately assessed and certified.

Universal indicator A chemical solution that changes colour to identify the strength of an acid or alkaline compound when it is immersed into it.

The resulting colour is matched against a shade chart to measure/gauge the exact pH level.

V

Valid tender A method of payment that is acceptable to the salon. Valid tender from a client paying for services could be cash, debit card, credit card, cheque, voucher etc.

Velcro rollers Self-cling setting rollers for use on dry hair. They produce a softer curl effect than wet setting rollers.

Vellus hair The soft, downy hair found on the body.

Vented brush A parallel, flat brush with a double row of rigid, plastic bristles (short and long) affixed to a brush head that is not solid. It is used for general brushing and straightening of short to mid-length hair.

Virgin hair Hair that has not been chemically treated.

Virus The smallest micro-organisms that cause infection and disease.

W

W/C Appointment abbreviation for wet cutting.

Warmth A reference to hair tones that appear golden, copper or red in colour.

Weave wind A perming technique for winding rods into the hair so that part of the mesh taken leaves hair out providing a multi-textured effect.

Wefts Long continuous strands of pre-coloured, pre-bonded hair that create a 'curtain' of hair that can be used to add to, or extend, a client's own natural hair.

Wetting agent A chemical agent that allows a liquid to spread more easily across or into a surface by lowering the liquid's surface tension.

Whorls A circular hair growth pattern that will influence or limit the styling options for a client, e.g. nape whorls.

Widow's peak A distinct point in the hairline in the centre of the forehead.

Workplace (Health Safety and Welfare) Regulations (1992) Regulations that stipulate that the employer is responsible for maintaining a safe, secure working environment that meets the needs of all employees.

Workplace policies This covers the documentation prepared by your employer on the procedures to be followed in your workplace.

Workplace practices Any activities, procedures, use of materials or equipment and working techniques used in carrying out your job.

Blended Learning Solutions for Hairdressing

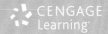

The Official Guides to Hairdressing at Level 1, 2 and 3 Textbooks by Leo Palladino and Martin Green

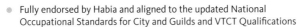

- Fully endorsed by Habia and aligned to the updated National Occupational Standards for City and Guilds and VTCT Qualifications

- This established series by bestselling authors Leo Palladino and Martin Green provides top quality pedagogy including exercises, activities, step-by-steps and illustrations to prepare students for the world of work

- The series works in perfect partnership with U2Learn and E-Teach Hairdressing ensuring a complete blended learning experience.

Lecturer Online Teaching Resources for Level 1, 2 and 3
E-Teach Hairdressing

www.eteachhairdressing.co.uk

- Content is linked directly to the *Official Guides to Hairdressing* textbooks at Level 1, 2 and 3

- Provides a host of PowerPoint presentations, handouts, interactive quizzes, activities and videos to bring the subject to life.

- The ready-made resources save on class preparation time and engage and motivate students.

Student Online Learning for Level 2 developed by Cengage Learning and Habia
U2Learn Hairdressing

U2Learn

- Content is linked directly to *Hairdressing: The Foundations Level 2* textbook.

- Provides a visual and engaging learning environment through games, exercises, animations and videos.

- Students can practice what they have learned and improve their knowledge retention.

For more information about our blended learning solutions for hairdressing please contact emea.fesales@cengage.com

HAIRDRESSING AND BEAUTY INDUSTRY AUTHORITY SERIES

Student Hairdressing textbooks

Begin Hairdressing: The Official Guide to Level 1 REVISED 2e *Martin Green*

Hairdressing – The Foundations: The Official Guide to Level 2 REVISED 6e *Leo Palladino and Martin Green*

Professional Hairdressing: The Official Guide to Level 3 REVISED 6e *Martin Green and Leo Palladino*

The Official Guide to the City & Guilds Certificate in Salon Service 1e *John Armstrong with Anita Crosland, Martin Green and Lorraine Nordmann*

The Colour Book: The Official Guide to Colour for NVQ Levels 2 and 3 1e *Tracey Lloyd with Christine McMillan-Bodell*

eXtensions: The Official Guide to Hair Extensions 1e *Theresa Bullock*

Salon Management *Martin Green*

Men's Hairdressing: Traditional and Modern Barbering 2e *Maurice Lister*

African-Caribbean Hairdressing 2e *Sandra Gittens*

The World of Hair Colour 1e *John Gray*

The Cutting Book: The Official Guide to Cutting at S/NVQ Levels 2 and 3 *Jane Goldsbro and Elaine White*

Professional Hairdressing titles

Trevor Sorbie: The Bridal Hair Book 1e *Trevor Sorbie and Jacki Wadeson*

The Art of Dressing Long Hair 1e *Guy Kremer and Jacki Wadeson*

Patrick Cameron: Dressing Long Hair 1e *Patrick Cameron and Jacki Wadeson*

Patrick Cameron: Dressing Long Hair 2 1e *Patrick Cameron and Jacki Wadeson*

Bridal Hair 1e *Pat Dixon and Jacki Wadeson*

Professional Men's Hairdressing: The art of cutting and styling 1e *Guy Kremer and Jacki Wadeson*

Essensuals, The Next Generation Toni and Guy: Step by Step 1e *Sacha Mascolo, Christian Mascolo and Stuart Wesson*

Mahogany Hairdressing: Step to Cutting, Colouring and Finishing Hair 1e *Martin Gannon and Richard Thompson*

Mahogany Hairdressing: Advanced Looks 1e *Martin Gannon and Richard Thompson*

The Total Look: The Style Guide for Hair and Make-up Professional 1e *Ian Mistlin*

Trevor Sorbie: Visions in Hair 1e *Trevor Sorbie, Kris Sorbie and Jacki Wadeson*

The Art of Hair Colouring 1e *David Adams and Jacki Wadeson*

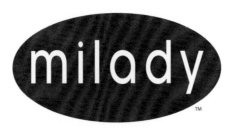

A part of Cengage Learning

For more than 80 years, Milady has been the number one provider for hair and beauty learning solutions and has provided the beauty industry with superior educational and professional learning materials. Spanning six continents, Milady has aided more than 10 million beauty professionals.

Milady also supports the salon and spa industry through personal consultation, business and life coaching, comprehensive organizational training and programs to assist salon and spa business owners to develop successful businesses.

Milady's range of successful textbooks includes Milady Standard Cosmetology 2012 Metric edition, Milady Standard Nail Technology 6th edition and Milady's Standard Professional Barbering, 5th edition.

For further information on Milady and Milady products please visit http://fe.cengage.co.uk/